Book

of

Sayings

PETA ZAFIR

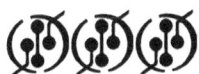

BOOK
OF
SAYINGS

Book 2

Peta Zafir Publishing
www.petazafir.com

ISBN 978-0-6452140-4-8

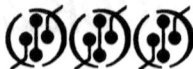

Peta Zafir Publishing
www.petazafir.com
Peta Zafir You Tube Channel

BOOKS BY PETA ZAFIR

Health in Poetry Book 1
Health in Poetry Book 2
Book of Sayings Book 1
Book of Sayings Book 2
Book of Sayings Book 3
Book of Sayings Book 4
Scenar For Beginners

All books are available in print and eBook format from:
www.petazafir.com/books

Dedication

I dedicate this book to my eldest son, Tyrone, who taught me how to be a mother and allowed me to grow up as a person, 15 minutes at a time. I have had the privilege to watch him grow into a man of strong conviction, high principles, determination and dedication.

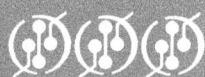

Adults understand the Consequences of their behaviour

and

Take responsibility for their actions

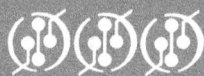

Before you Act

Think, Consider and Understand

what is pushing your behaviour and

Make choices from Love

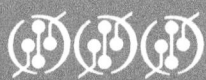

Nourish your body
with healthy clean food
Nourish your mind
with positive thoughts
Nourish your energy
with rest and contentment
Nourish your spirit
with reflection and contemplation

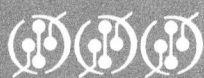

What we eat

Nourishes our bodies, energy and spirit

Stay conscious, be present

You are worth the best

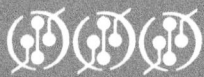

Turmoil and tribulations
can be painful and disruptive
Cull those people that are
aggressive, jealous and destructive
They are on their own journey

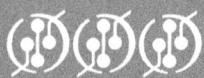

Walk through life with
self-caring and love

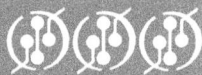

Find Strength in your Conviction

Calm in your Decisions

Peace in your Love and

Serenity in your Silence

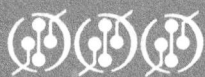

Life holds lessons to be learned

Challenges to be overcome

Joys to be experienced

And a future of awareness

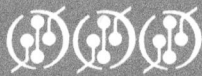

Become clear about
the person you want to be
The life you want to live
The people you want around you and
The future you want to create

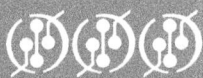

Passion will illuminate your Path

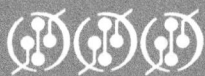

Try your hardest

Work your best

Compete your strongest

Perform your highest and

Be the BEST YOU that YOU can be

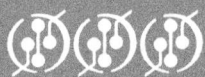

You are Enough

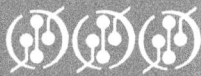

The only thing in life you need to ask is

Did you do your best

the rest is left to chance

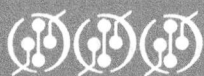

Do not judge yourself on the outcome only on the input

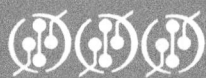

Find

The Family who will nourish you

The Home that brings you peace

The Work that fires your passion

The Friends that offer you support

The Partner who gives unconditional love

And a Life lived in harmony and serenity

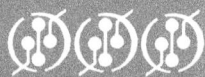

Money may offer Choice

however

Money does not offer Fulfilment

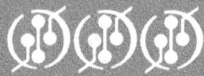

Your responsibility in this life
is to understand that you are a most amazing
unique, special and talented person alive
and only you have your gifts

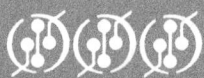

Opportunities come

when you work hard towards your goals

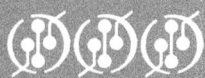

You are worth unconditional love

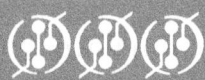

You do not have to criticize yourself

You do not have to judge yourself

You do not have to understand others

Just be the best you that you can be

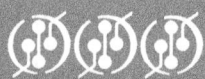

Aim high and reach the pinnacle of your success

happiness and health

YOU are worth it

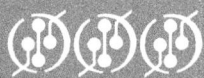

Do not judge yourself

Do not compare yourself

Do not question your uniqueness

Work through the process and

Hope will present the positive Path

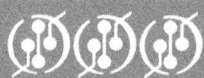

Walk into each day with a new open heart

feel the love and take the chances

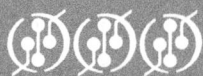

Go out today and live a full life

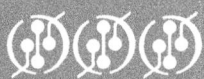

All consequences are learning

All decisions are learning

All results are learning

There are no failures

Just lessons learnt

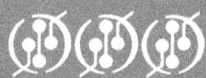

Promote Protect and Respect

Do not Abuse and Misuse

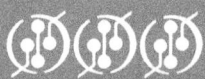

Age is only a number

It does not stop you

You stop you

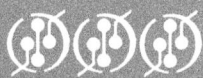

Start today

Do a little more each day

Learn something new

Begin with small steps

Add some determination and

Everything is Possible

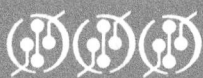

Every day is a day closer

to a brighter

happier and more serene path

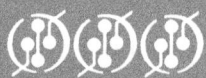

Don't let society's idea of Age

Determine who you are and

What you are able to do

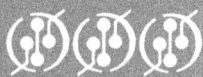

Hindsight is learning

What Choices did I make

What Steps did I take

What Decisions did I relate

What Path did I create

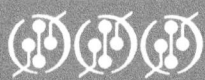

In understanding our Past

We learn and grow

And purify our Present

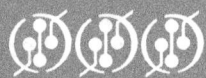

Do not let the fear of failure

Stop you today

Walk into each day anew

Trust yourself and make life Happen

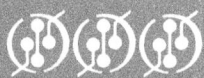

Make your life

More Loving, More Peaceful

More Honest, More Connected

More Adventurous, More Courageous

More Giving and More Fulfilling

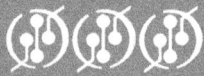

Find your inner strength

The ability to find the way

The determination to work through

The strength to never give up

The clarity to illuminate the Path

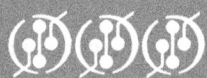

Your Vision is limited

only by your imagination

Your strength is limited

only by your determination

Your Spirit is limited

only by your connection to Universe

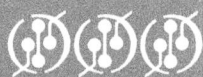

Life may appear unsurmountable

Clear away the debris

Make positive choices

Create health and

Live in Love and Peace

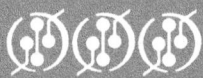

You can come through anything

if you want to

Give yourself time, Experience the pain

Strengthen your soul, Do the work

Be Honest with yourself

Keep getting up and

Keep moving forward

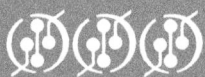

Just for Today

Live in the sunshine not in the shadows

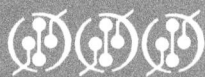

You are Important

Be Informed

Ask the questions

Understand the Process

Enquire about the Outcomes

You are worth it

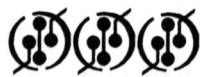

Peta Zafir Publishing

www.petazafir.com

Peta Zafir You Tube Channel

BOOKS BY PETA ZAFIR

Health in Poetry Book 1

Health in Poetry Book 2

Book of Sayings Book 1

Book of Sayings Book 2

Book of Sayings Book 3

Book of Sayings Book 4

Scenar For Beginners

All books are available in print and eBook format from:

www.petazafir.com/books

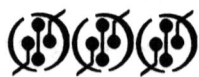